PLAY & LEARN
PAPERDOLL FRIENDS

Learn about the human body
with these anatomically-correct friends

By Cath Hakanson

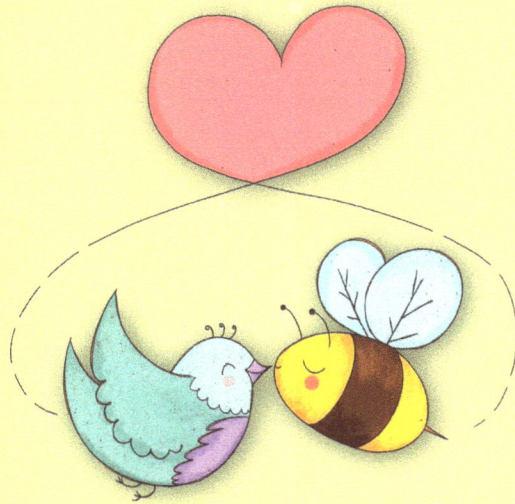

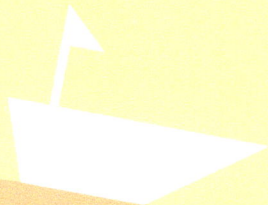

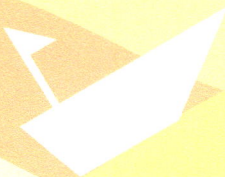

PLAY & LEARN
PAPERDOLL FRIENDS

by Cath Hakanson

Published by Sex Ed Rescue
PO Box 7903 | Cloisters Square WA 6850 | Australia

sexedrescue.com

This material represents the views, opinions and education of its author and has been produced with the intention that it acts purely as general information. It is not intended to be taken or used as a substitute for medical or other professional advice. We do not assume any responsibility for any liability, loss, damage or risk that may follow from the use or reliance of this material.

Dolls illustrated by Embla Granqvist
Clothing illustrated by Moch. Fajar Shobaru
Cover and interior design by Jevgenija Bitter

For permission contact:
cath@sexedrescue.com

ISBN-13: 978-0-6486900-9-2

INSTRUCTIONS

1. Color in the dolls and clothes before cutting out.

2. For best results, glue the doll to cardboard with a gluestick and allow to dry before cutting.

3. Carefully cut out dolls and stand with sharp scissors.

4. Cut along dotted line on both the stand and the doll base.

5. Insert the stand onto the base.

6. Cut out the clothes. Fold tabs over, slip tabs behind doll to fit. Clothes will fit all dolls.

TIP An alternative method to attach clothes (with no tabs) is to use Scotch® Restickable Strips. Attach half a sticky strip to the doll and clothes will be easy to change, with no more torn tabs and clothes!

FOR MORE HOURS OF IMAGINATIVE PLAY AND FUN, YOU CAN DOWNLOAD A FREE PRINTABLE PAPER HOUSE FOR YOUR DOLLS AT **https://sexedrescue.com/dollhouse/**

ALEX

If using clothes with tabs, cut between hair and shoulder so that tab for clothes will fit over shoulder.

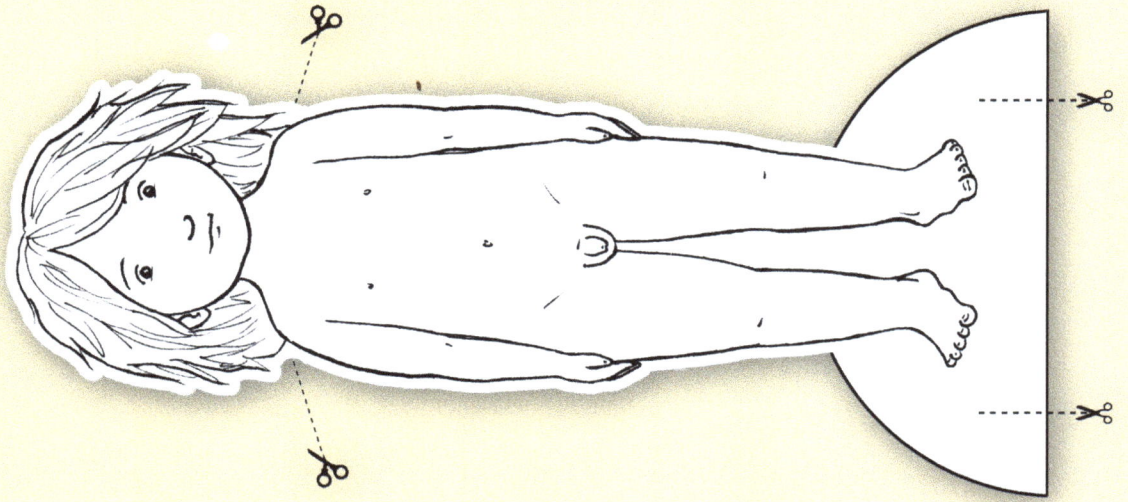

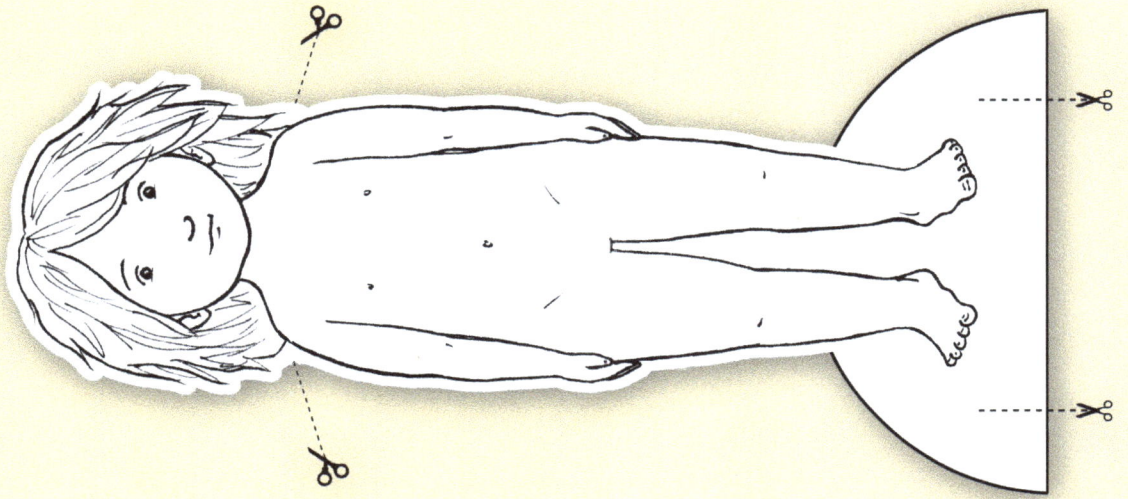

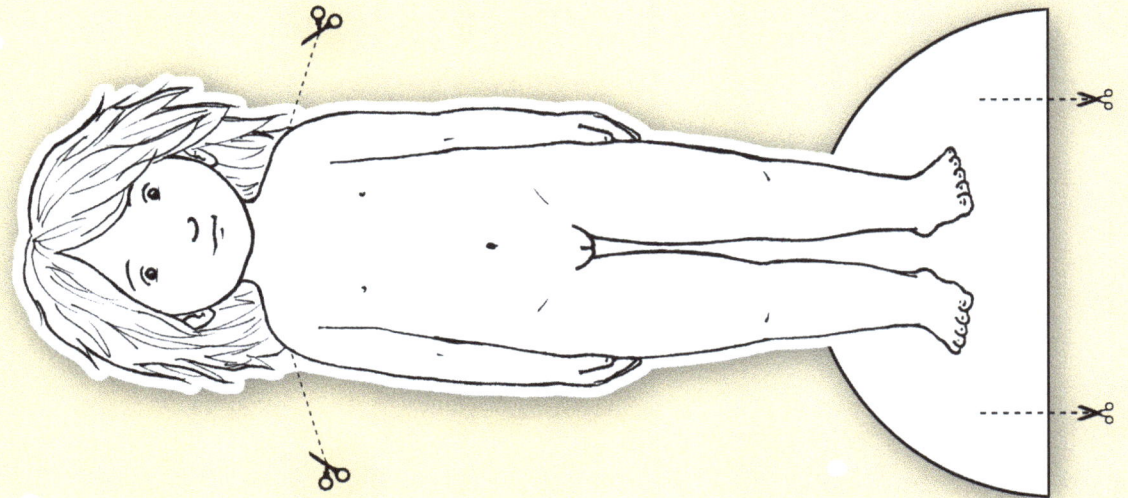

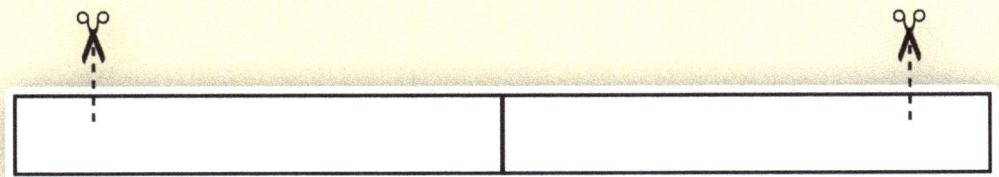

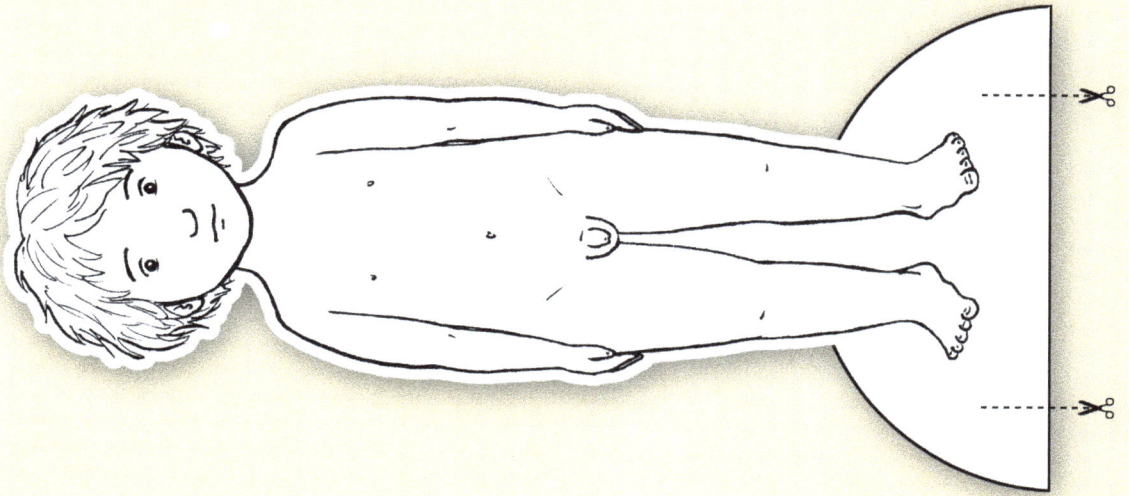
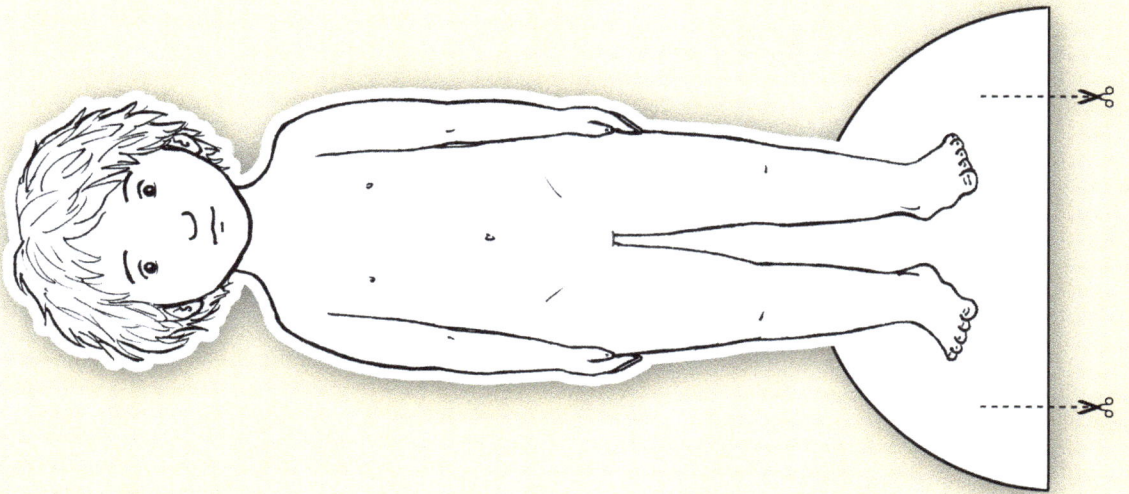
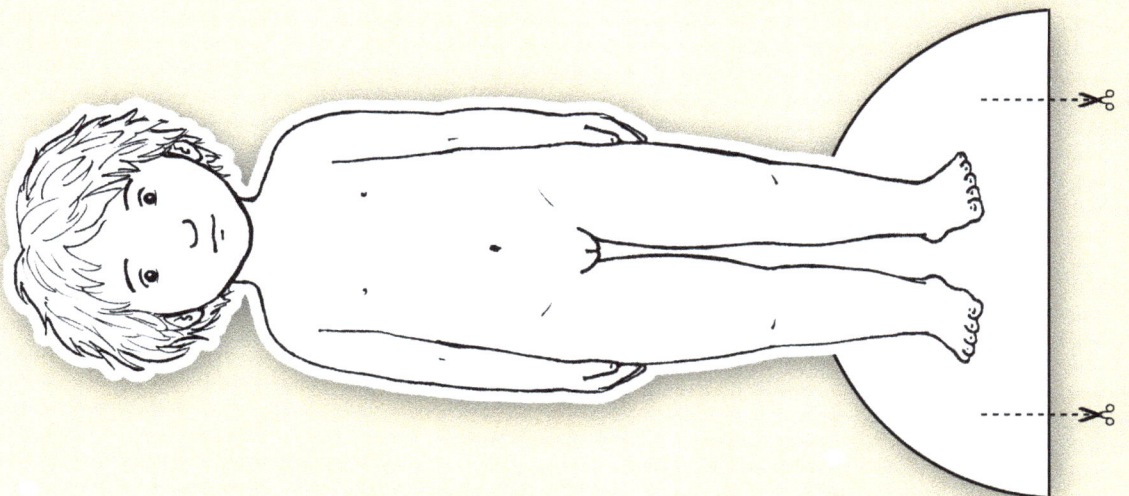

RILEY

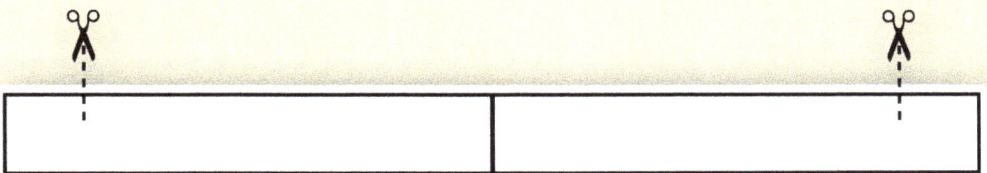

BAILEY

If using clothes with tabs, cut between hair and shoulder so that tab for clothes will fit over shoulder.

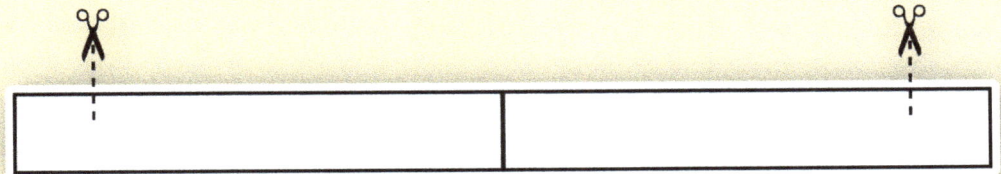

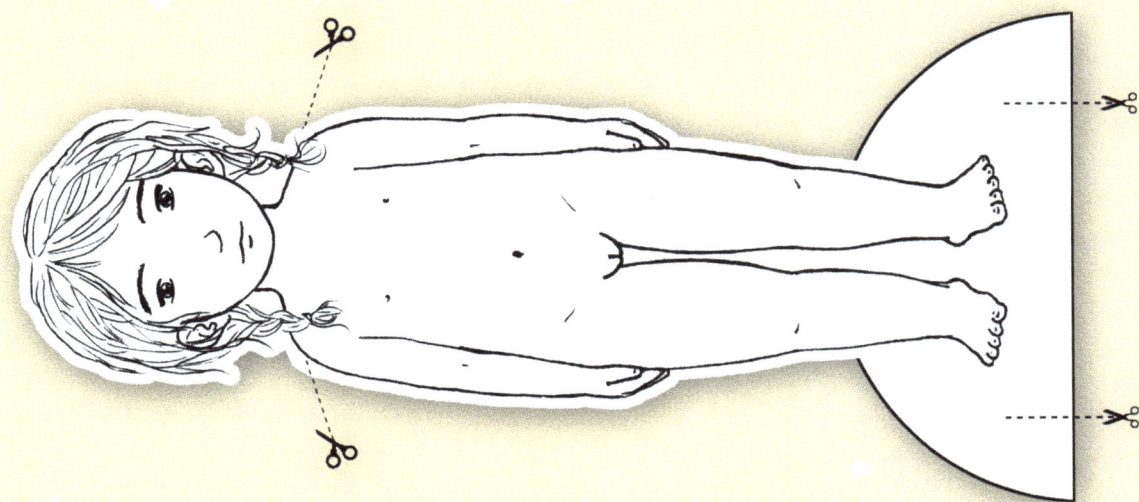

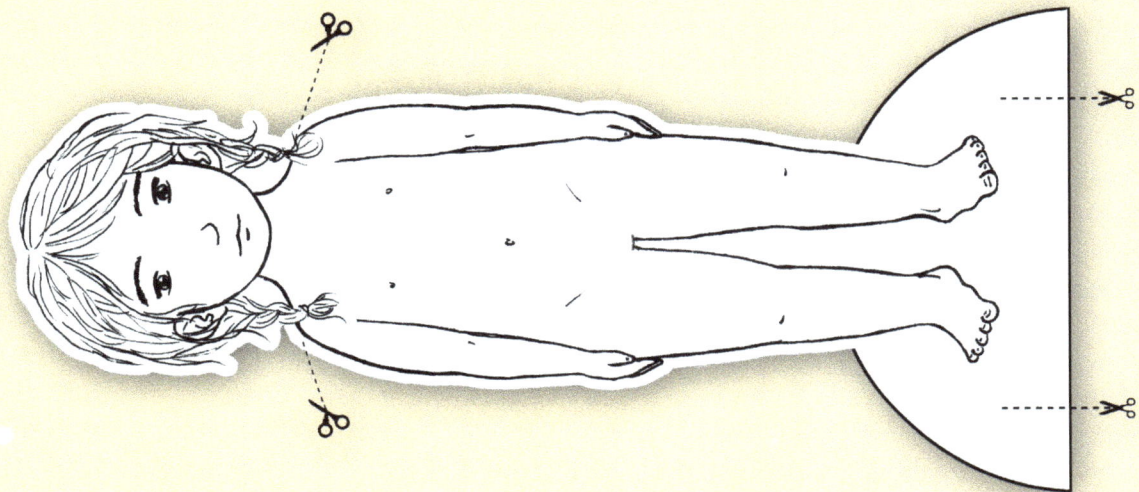

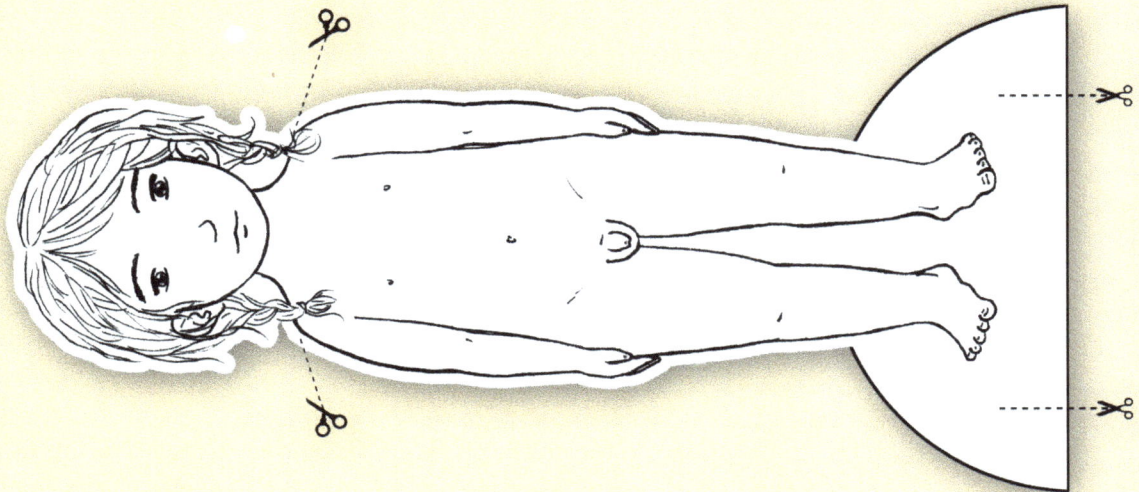

ASH

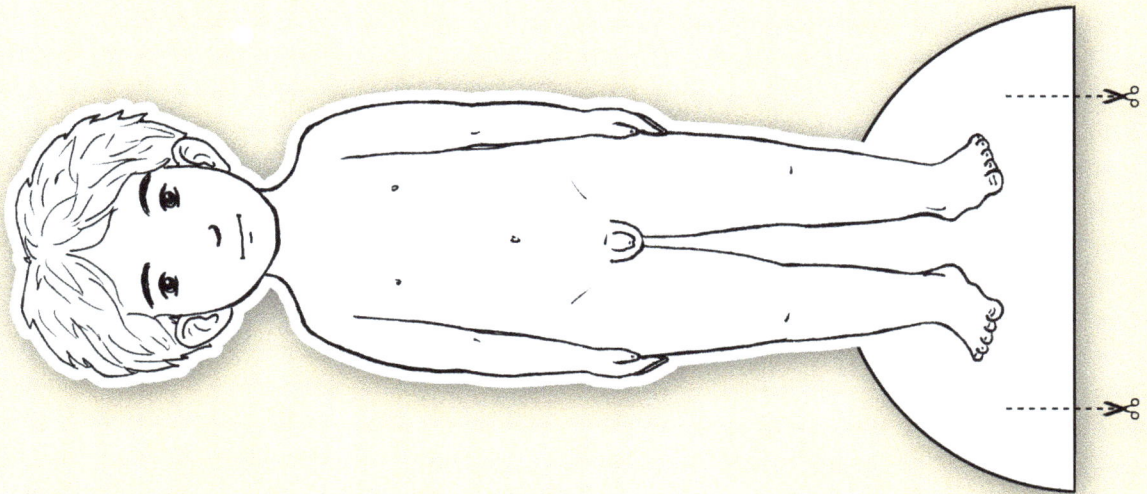

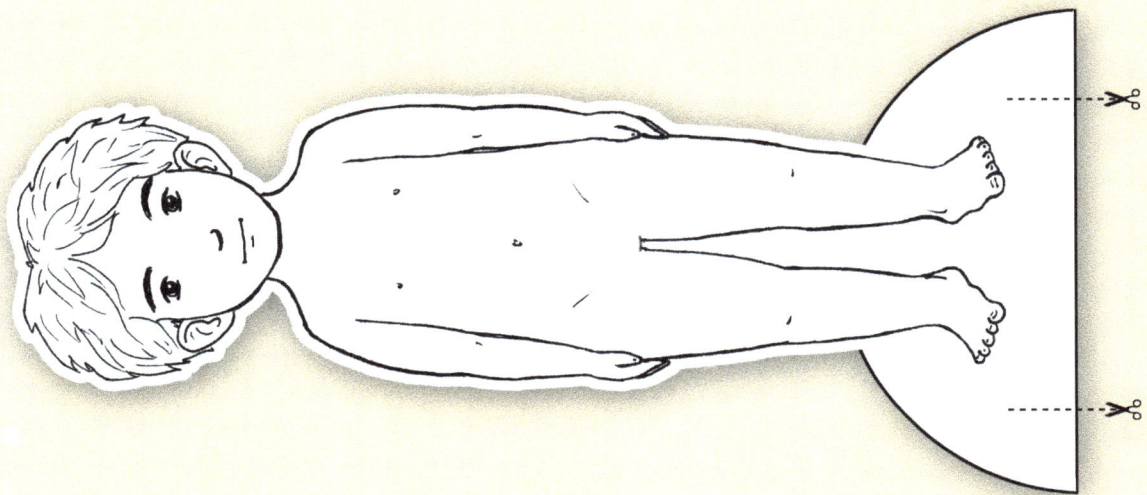

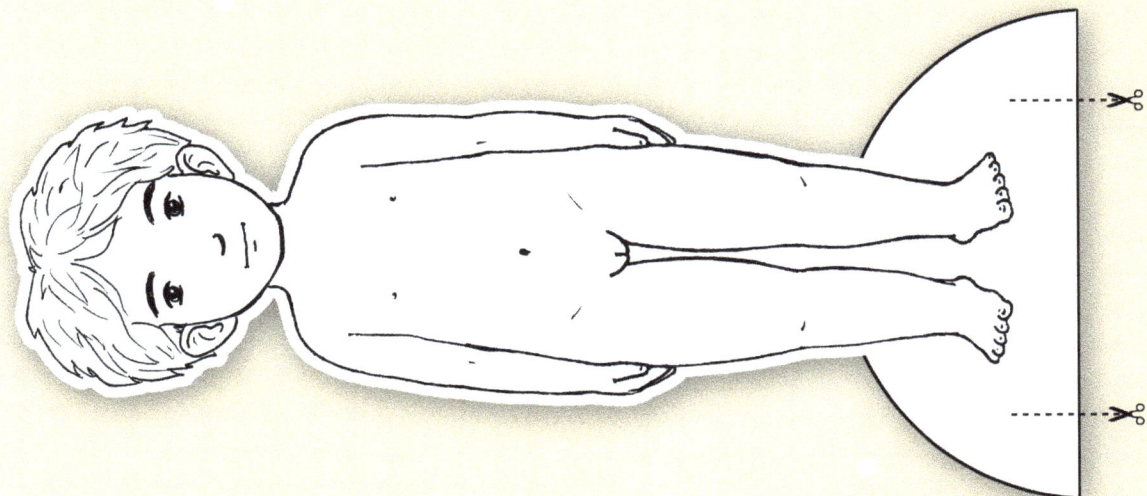

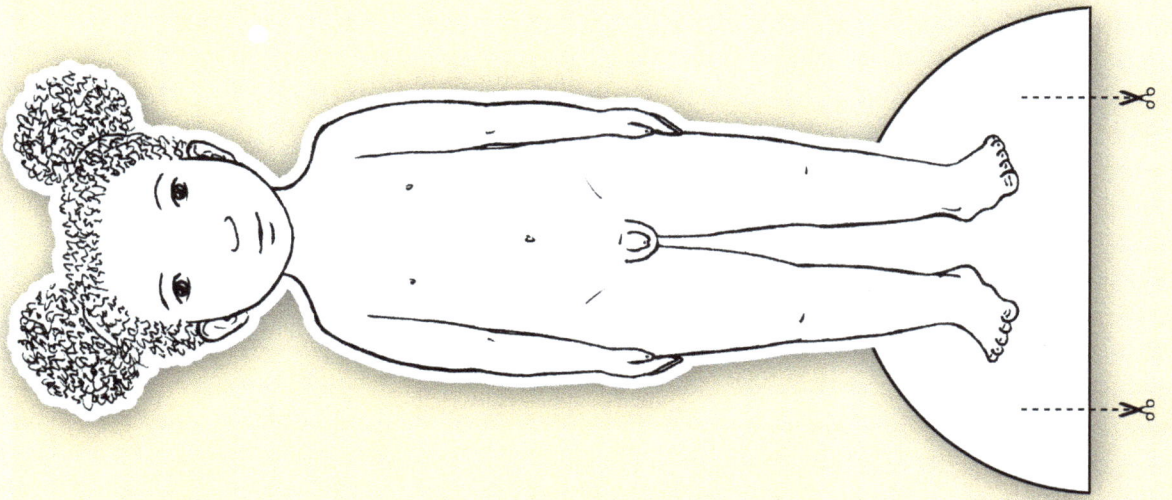

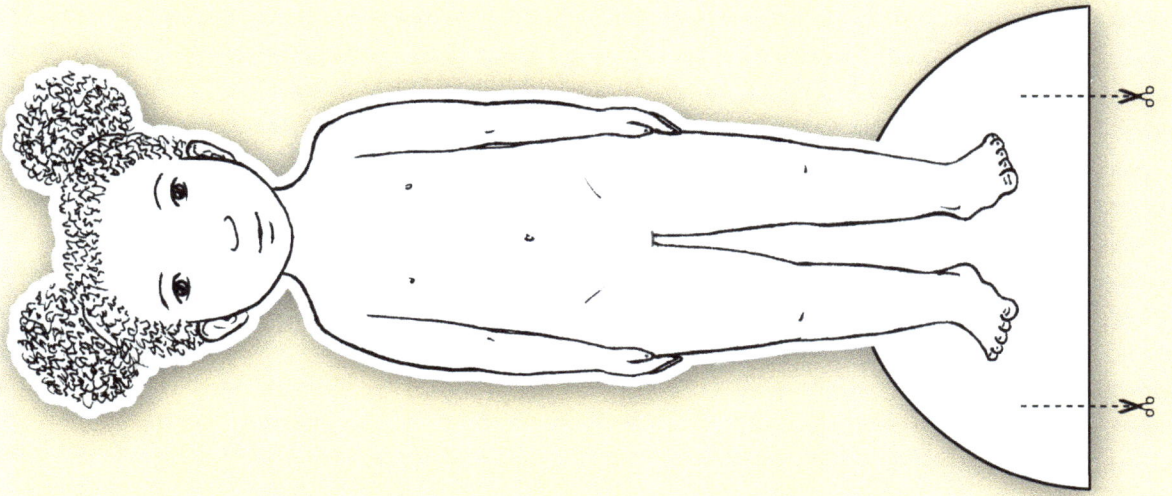

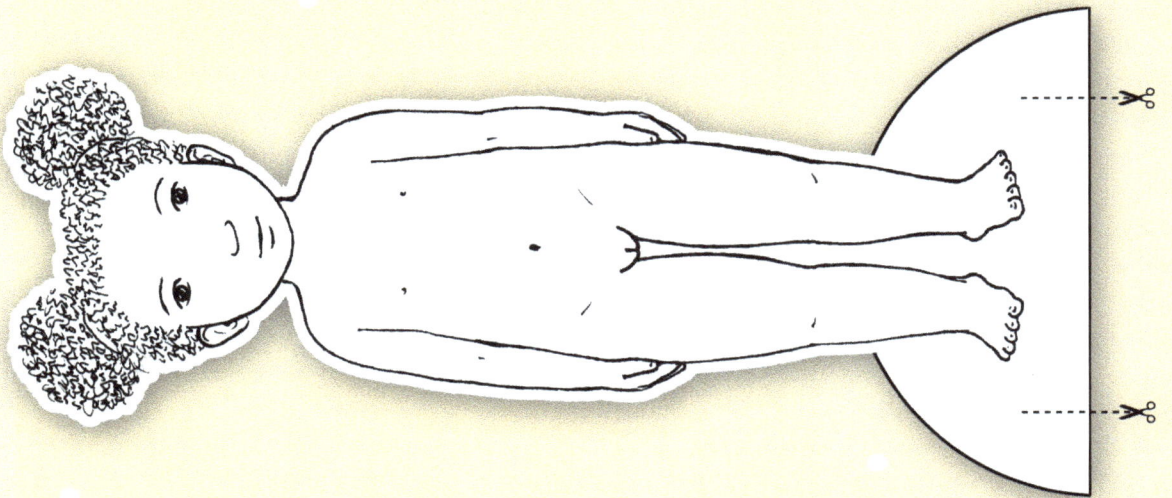

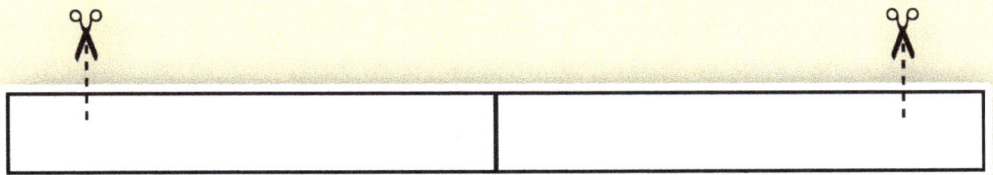

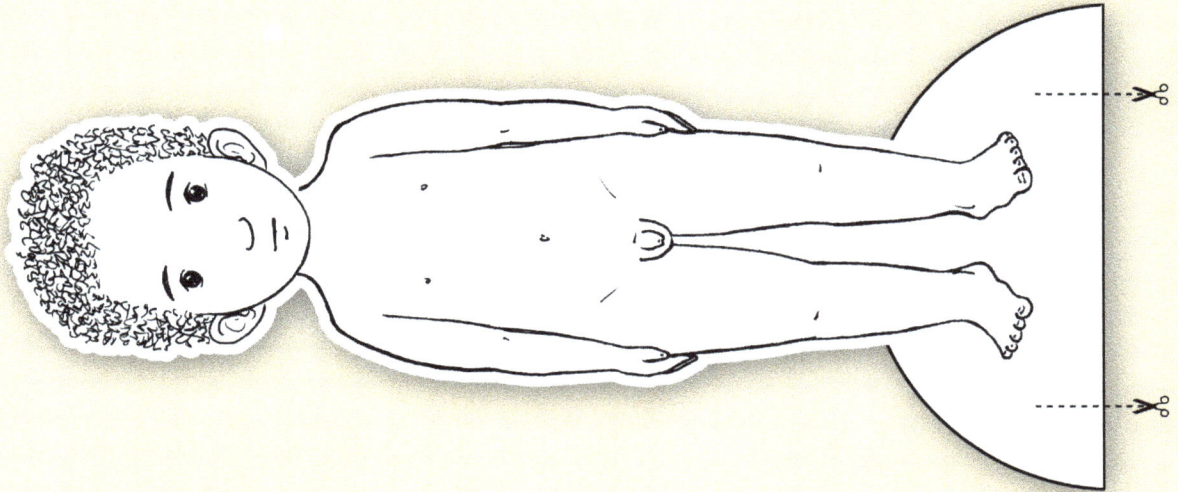

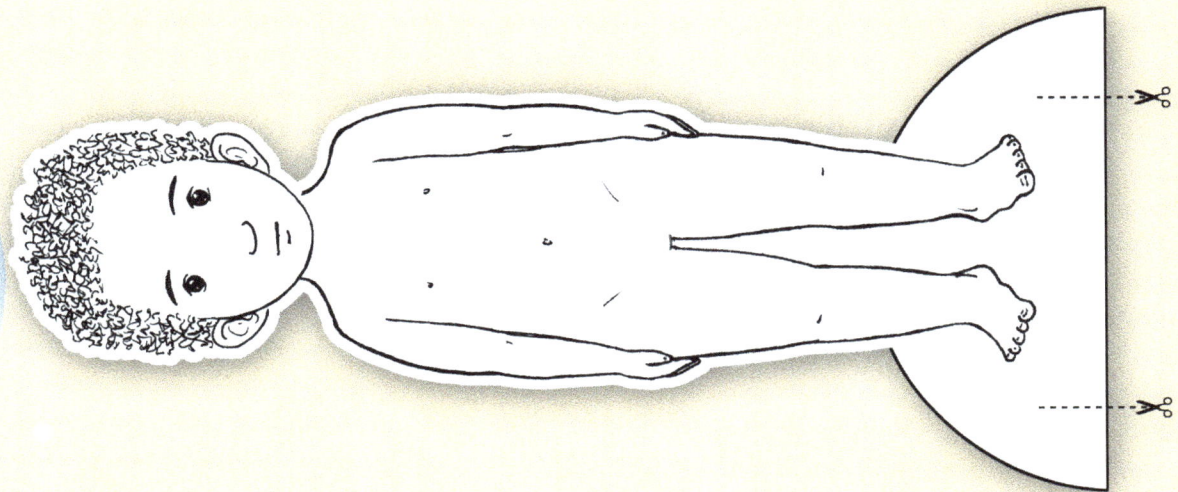

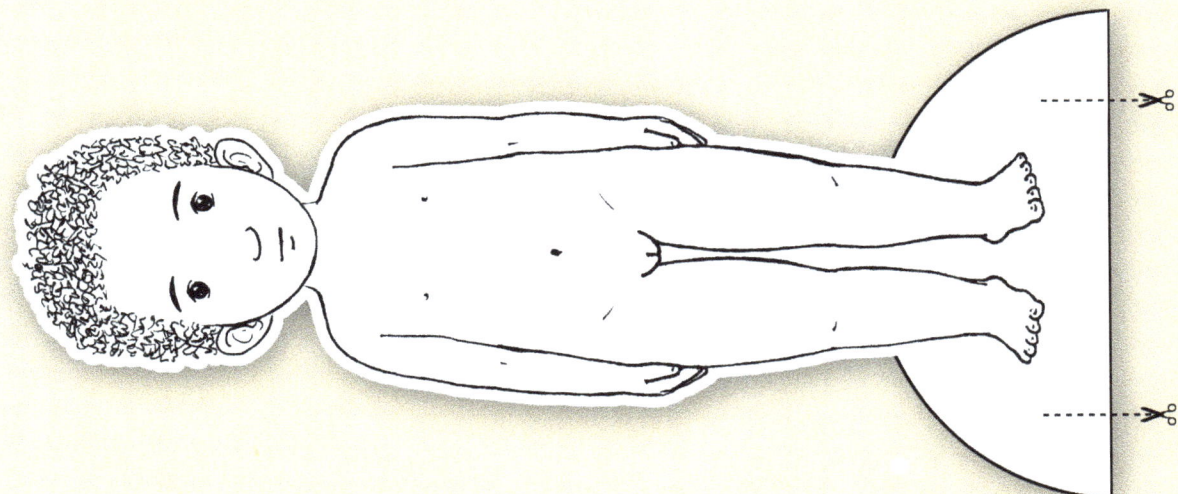

RORY

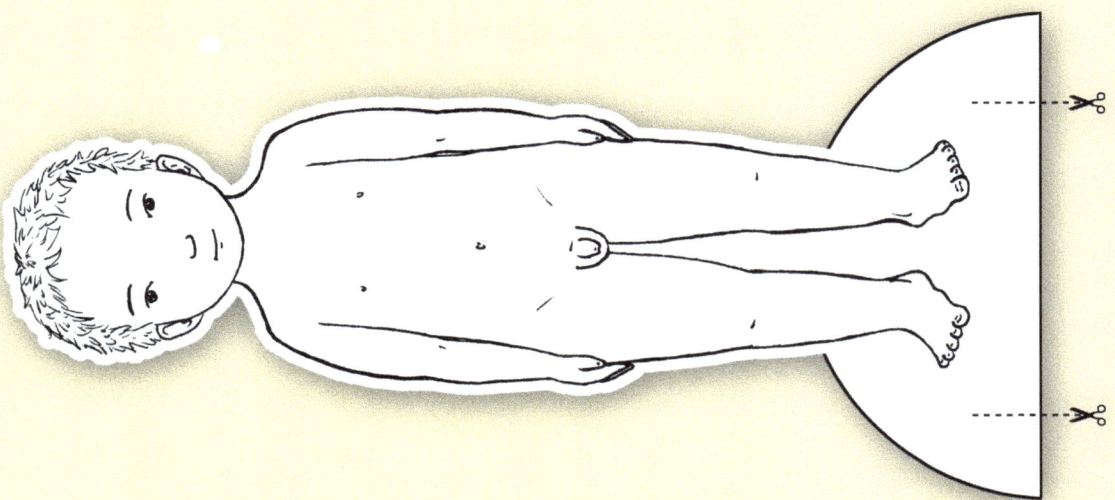

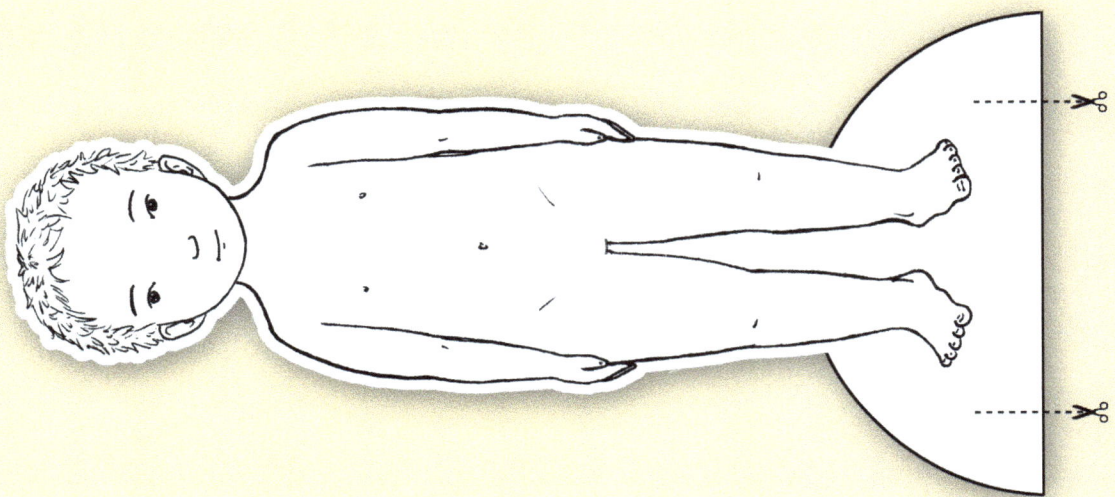

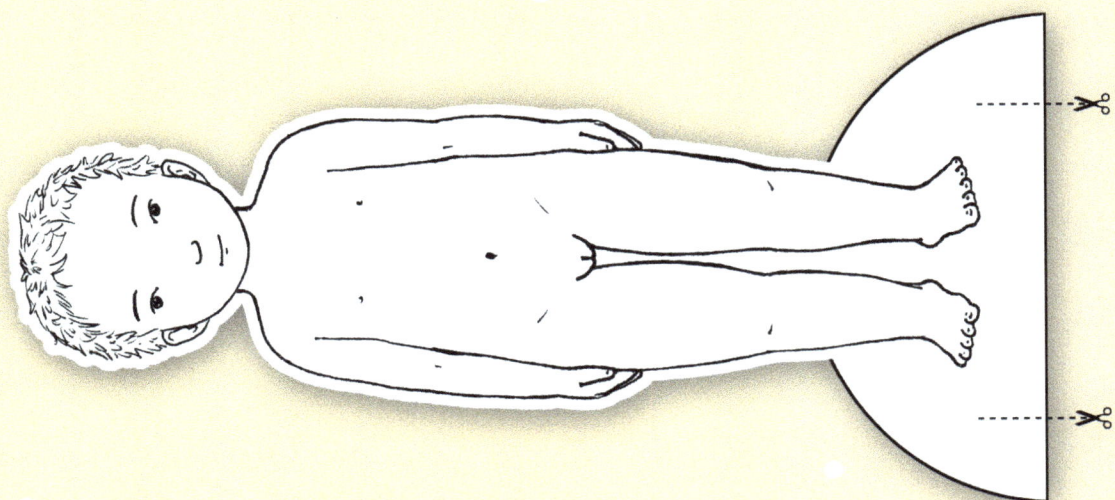

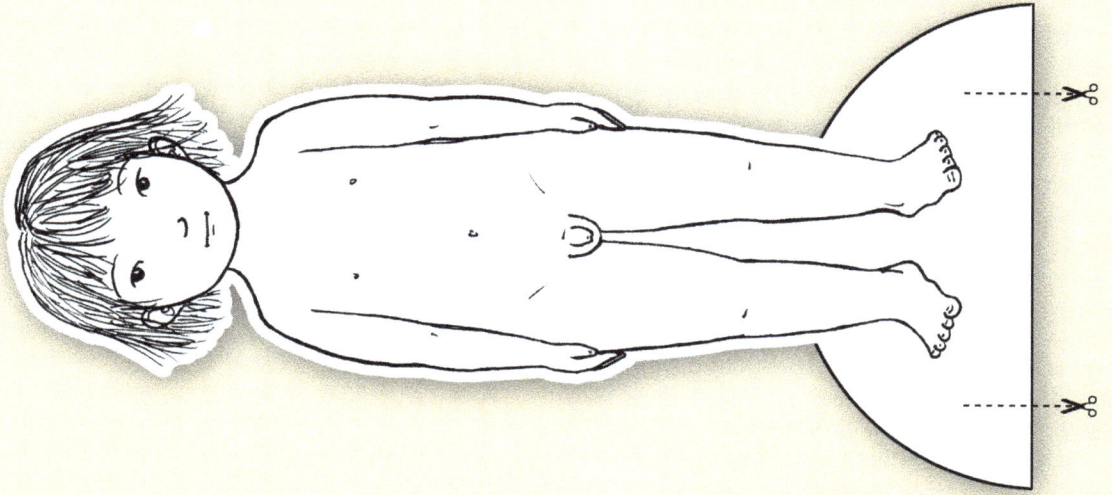

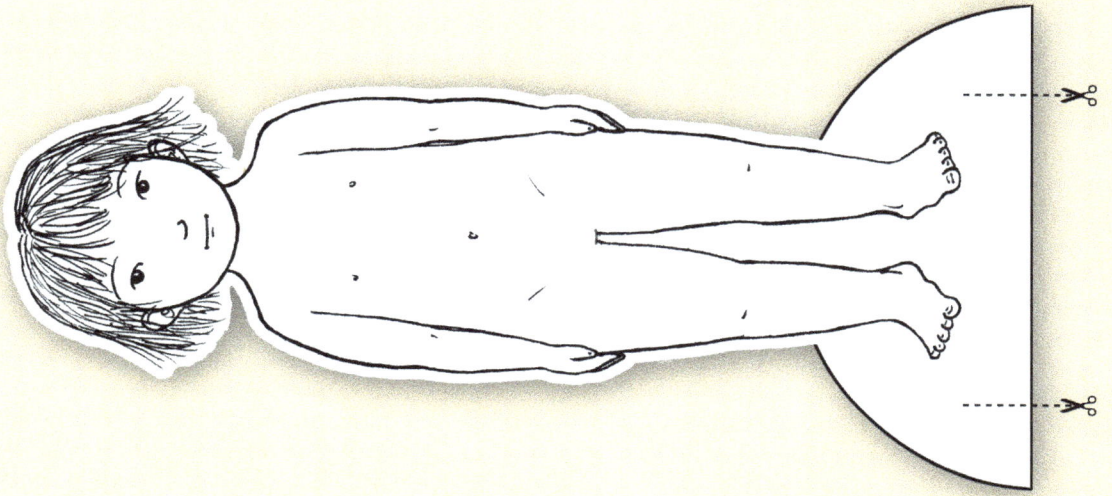

CHRIS

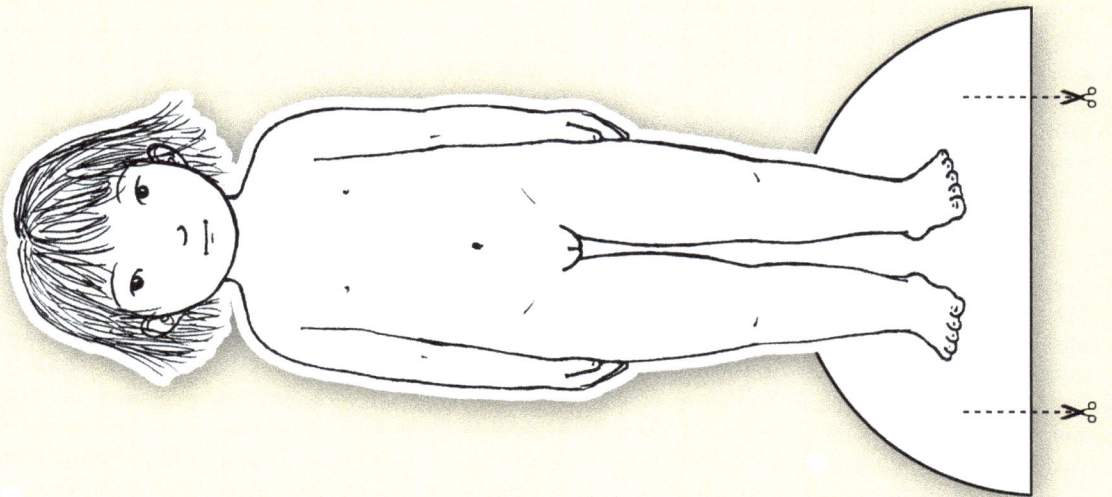

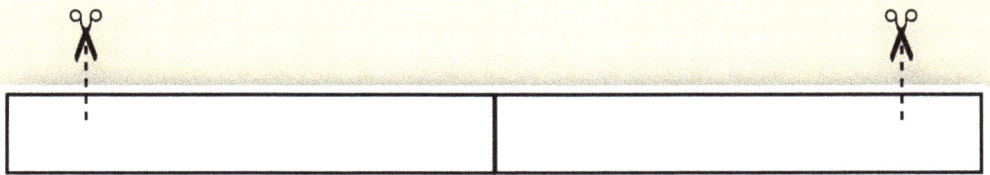

SASHA

If using clothes with tabs, cut between hair and shoulder so that tab for clothes will fit over shoulder.

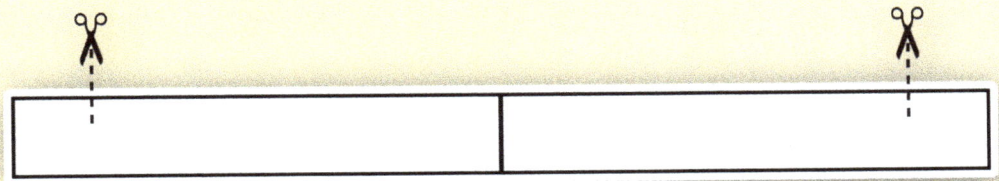

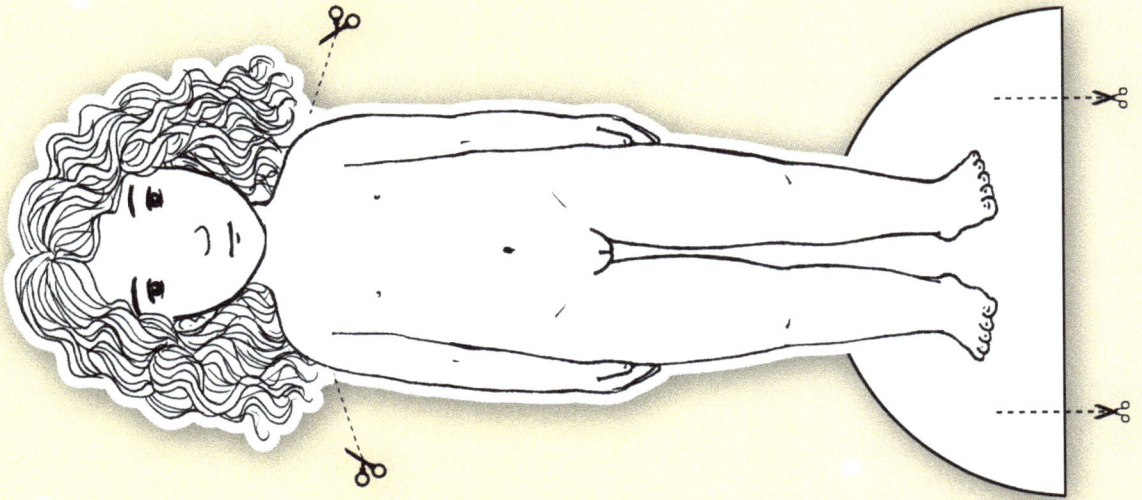

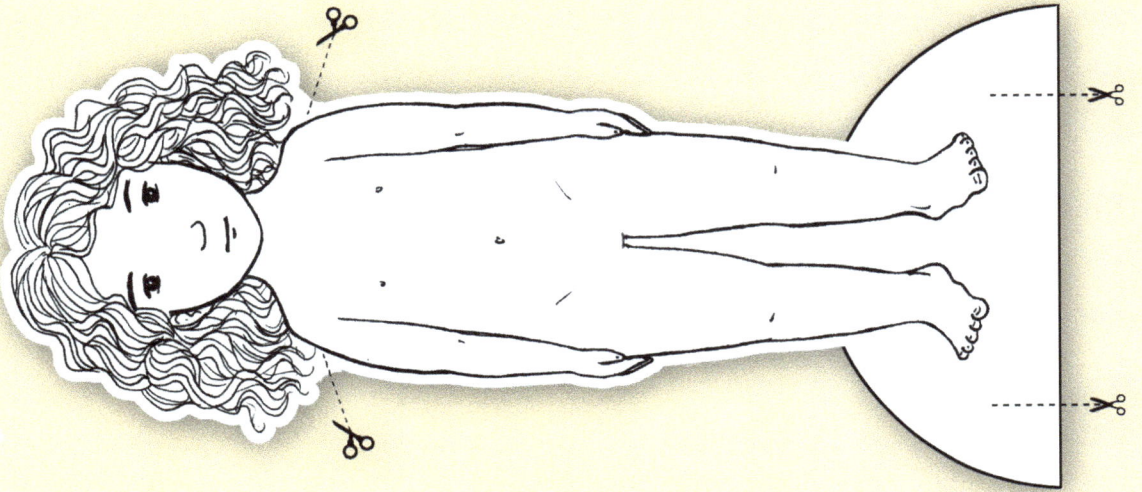

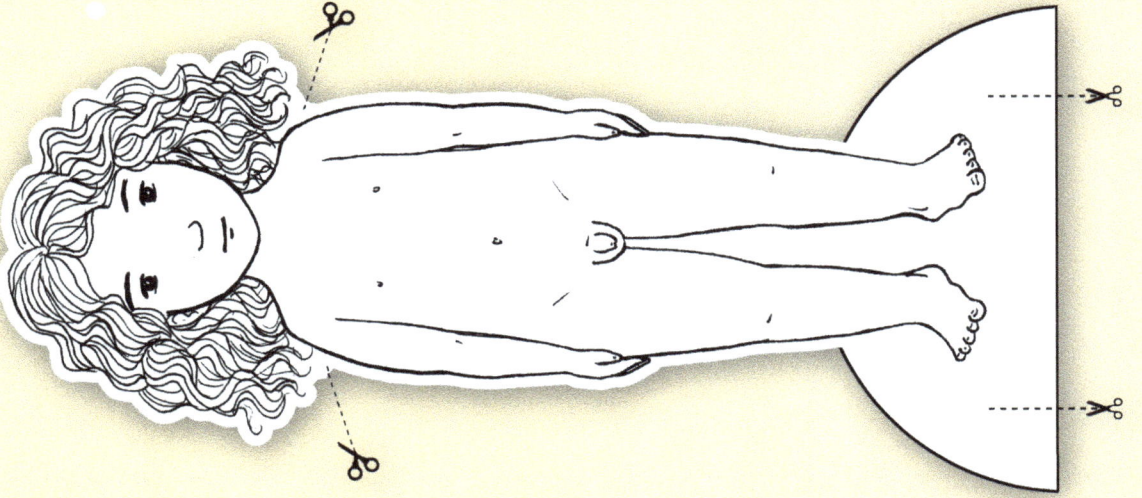

REECE

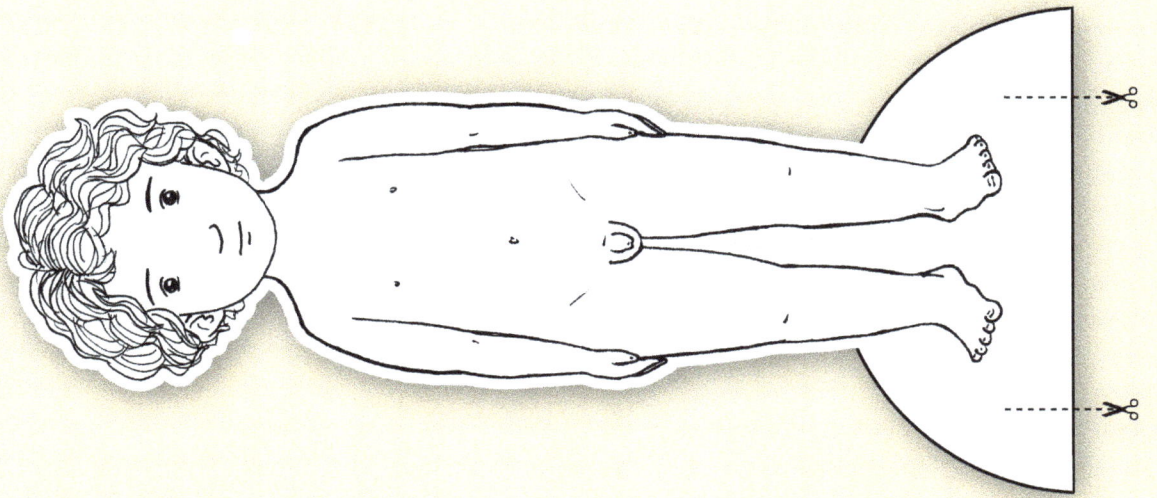

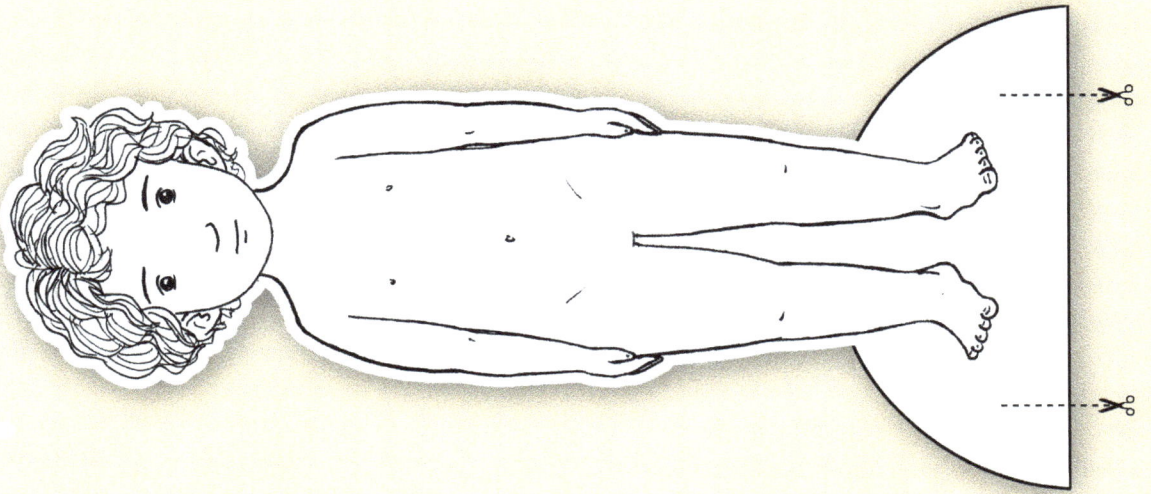

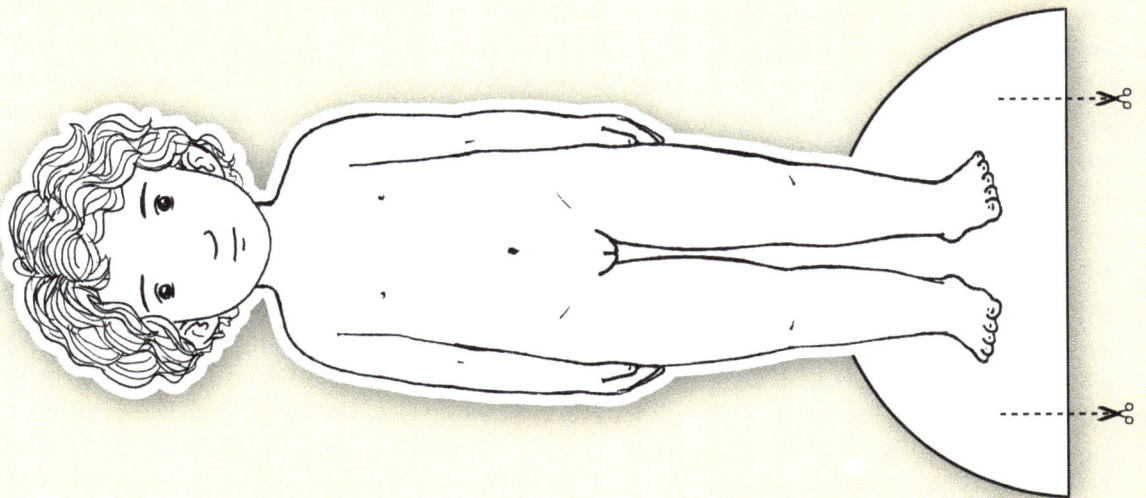

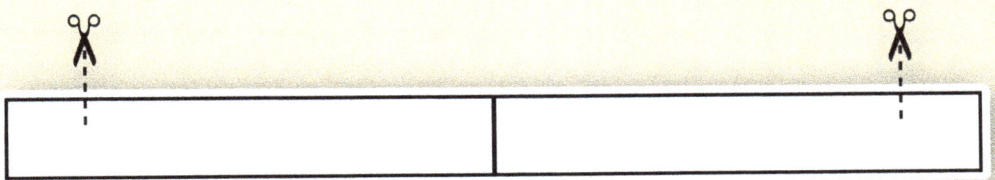

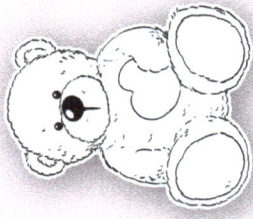

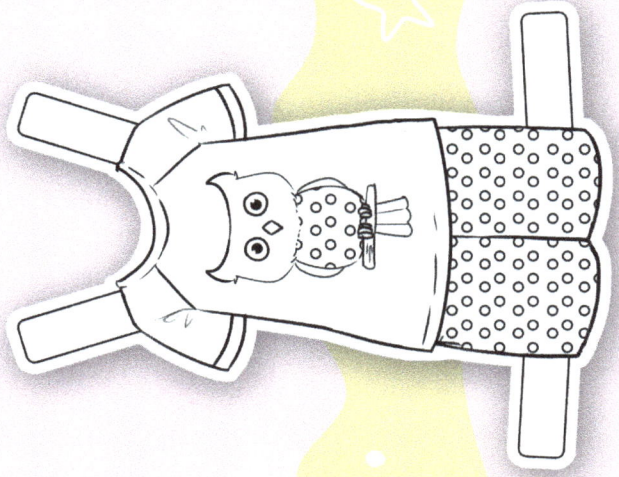

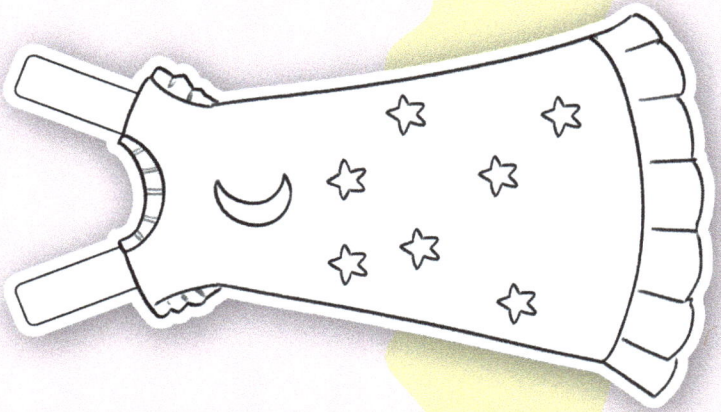

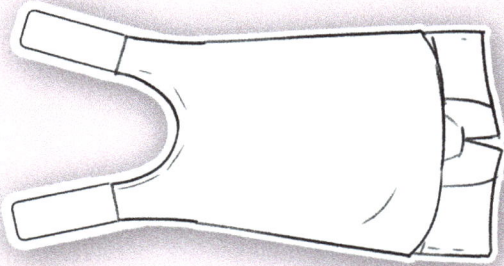

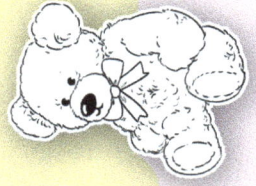

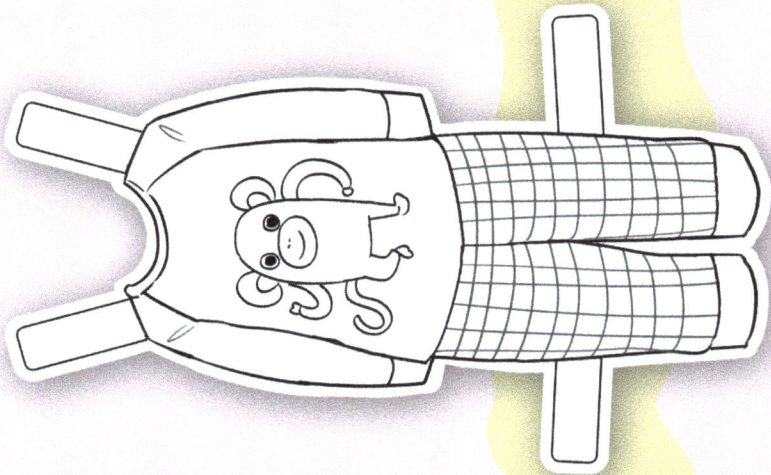

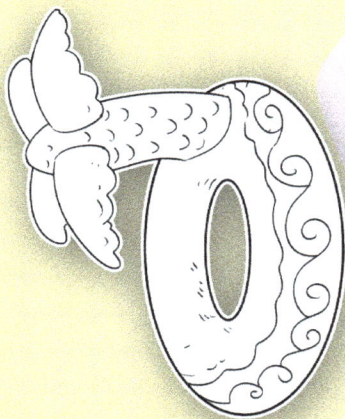

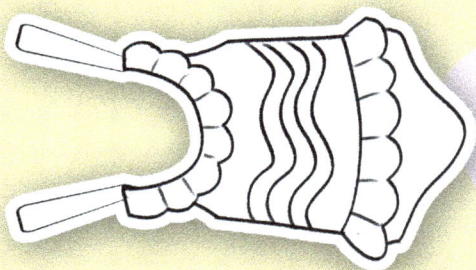

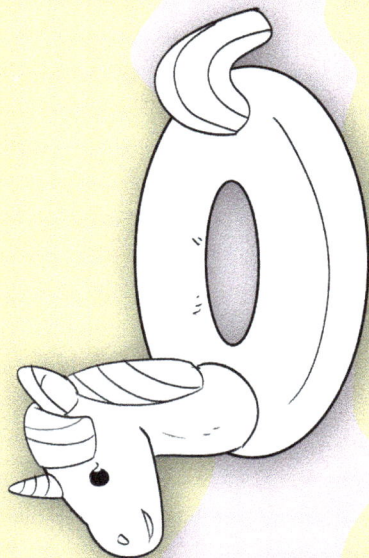

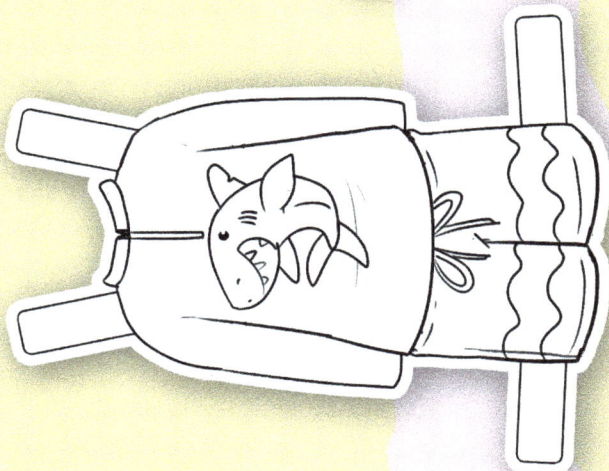

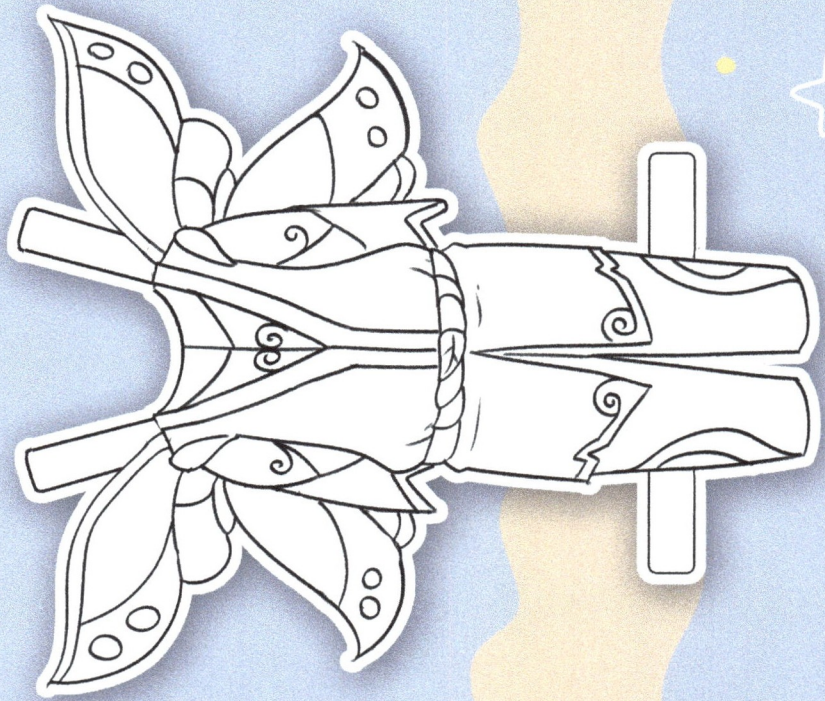

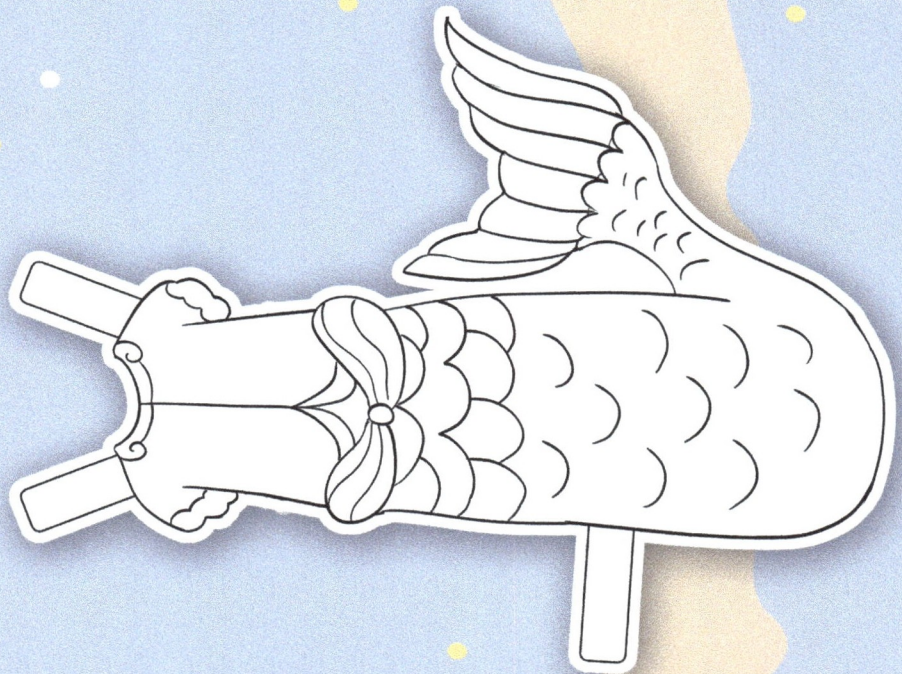

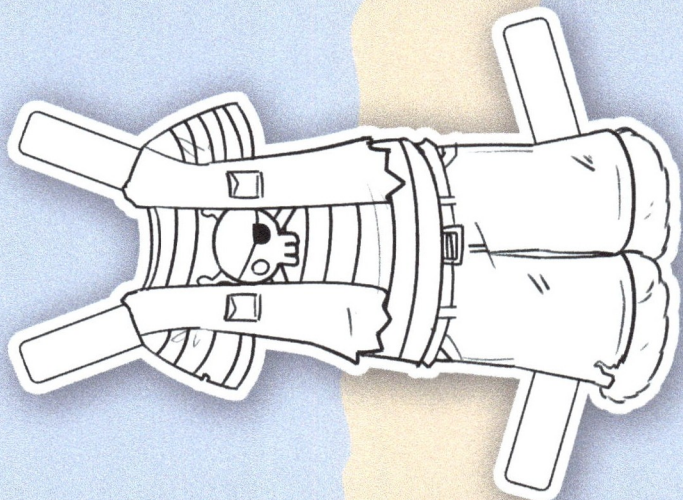

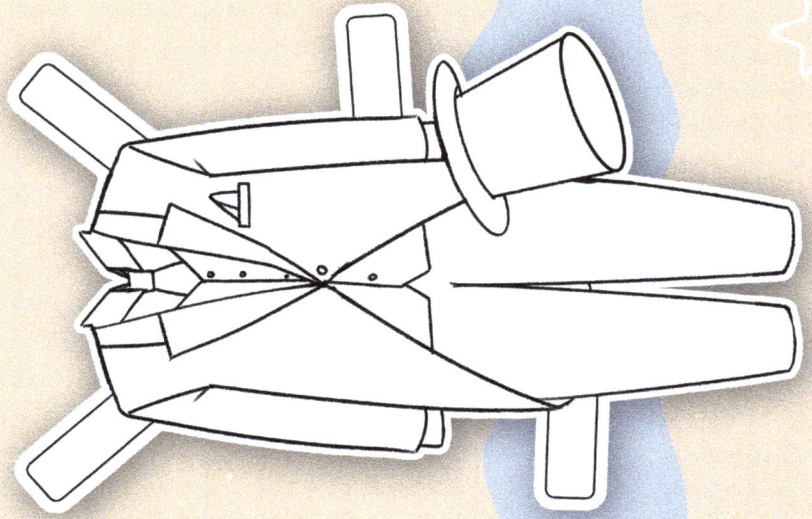

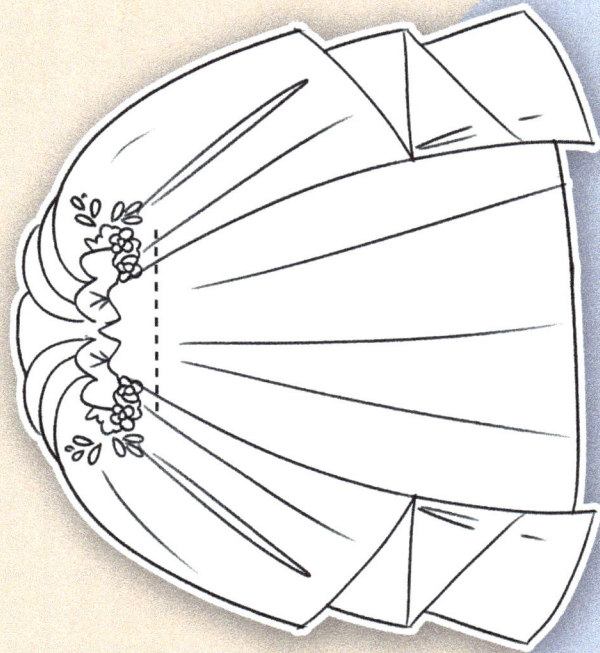

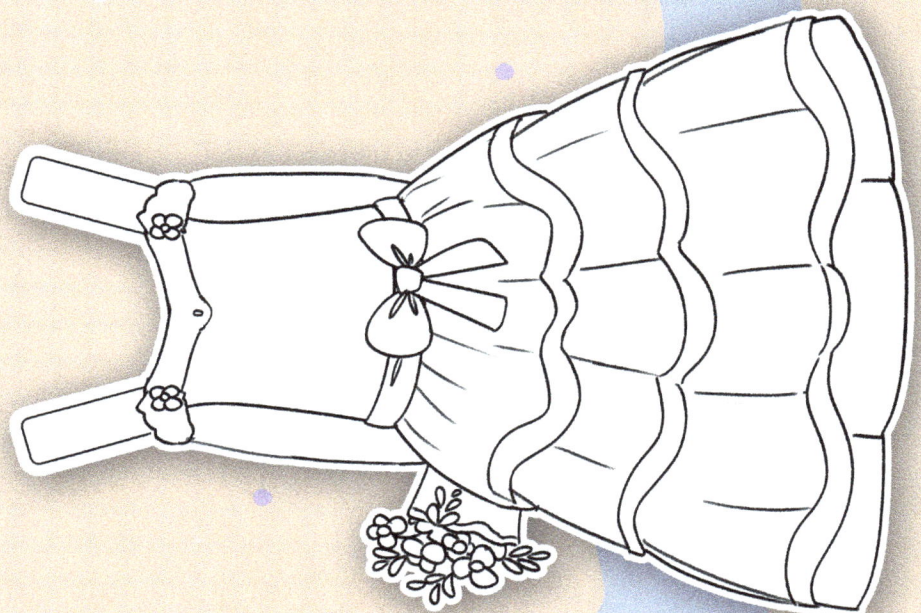

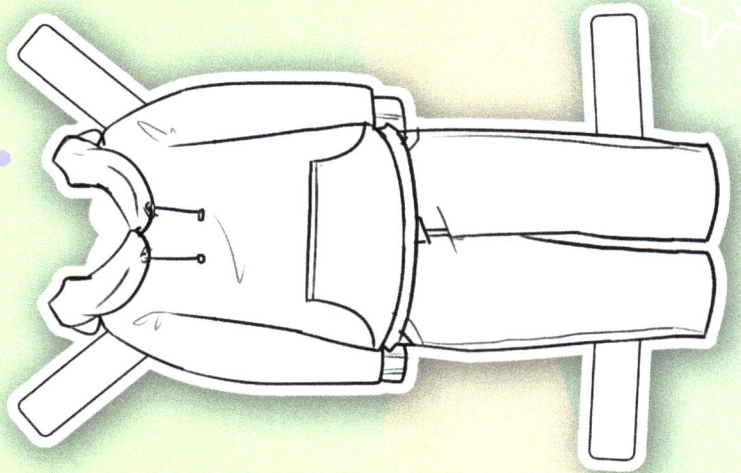

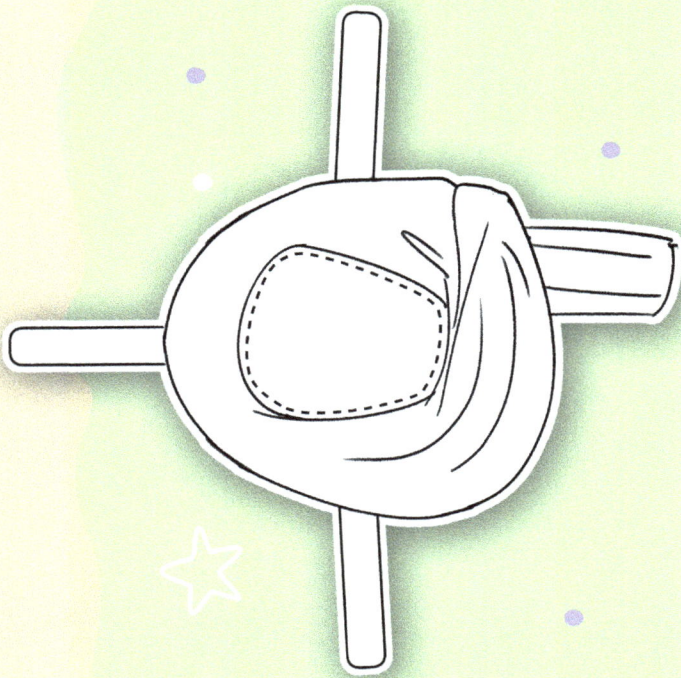

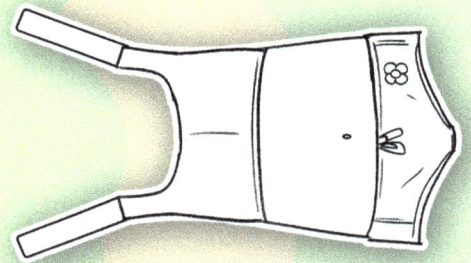

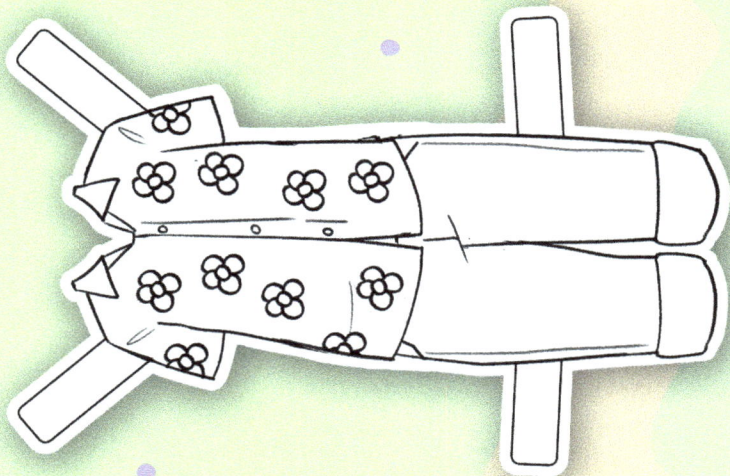

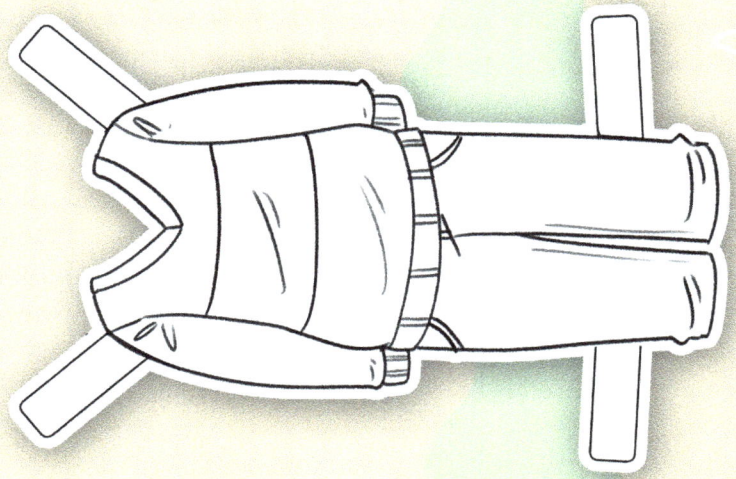

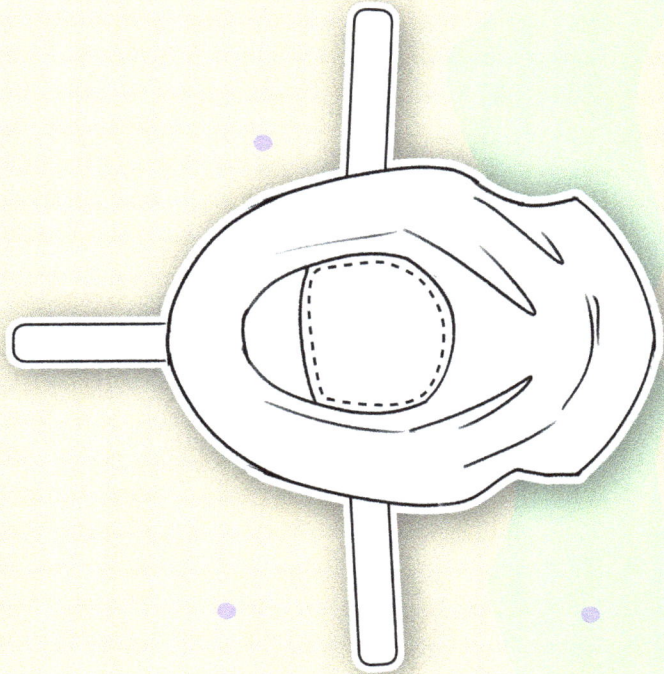

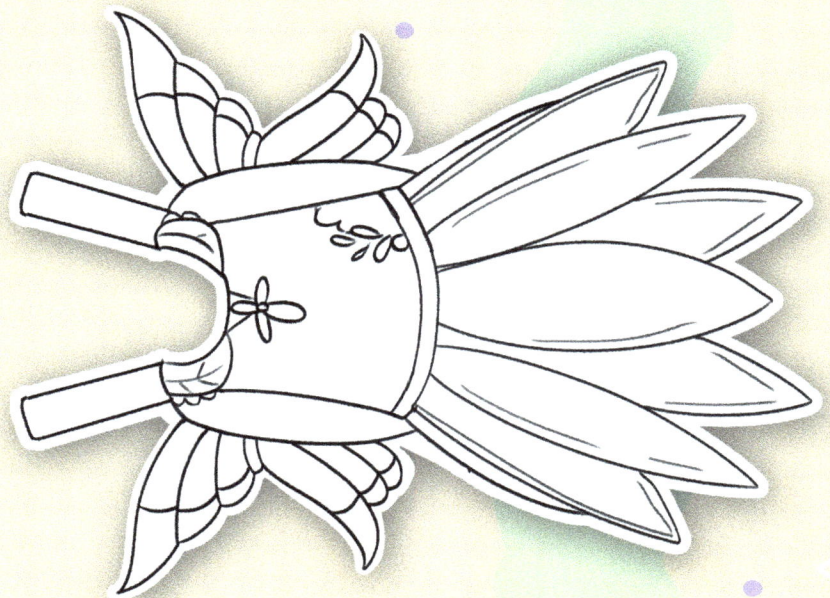

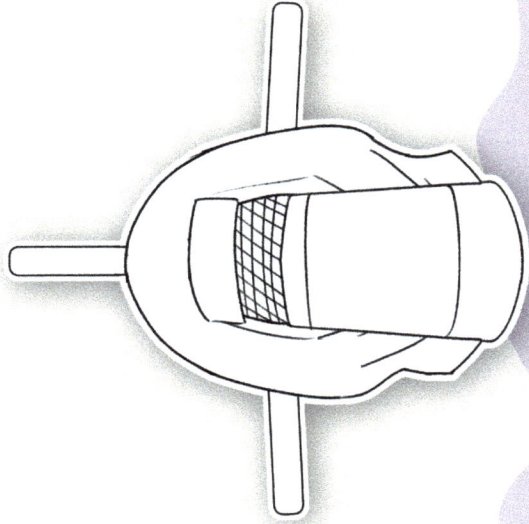

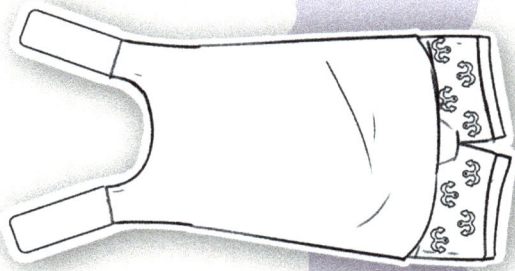

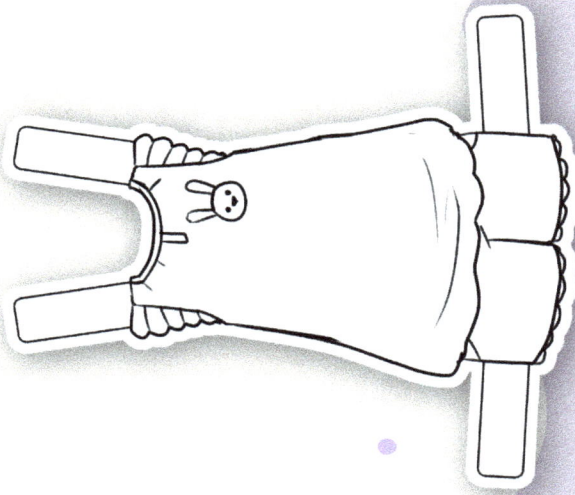

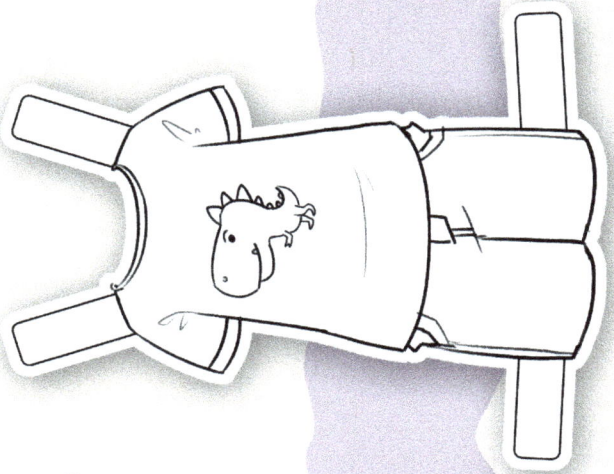

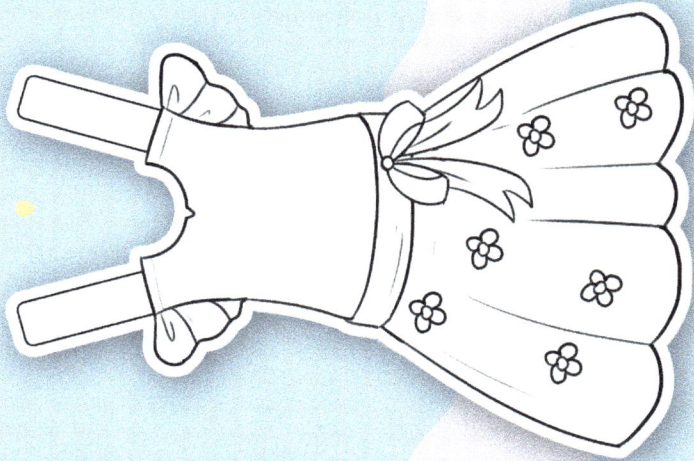

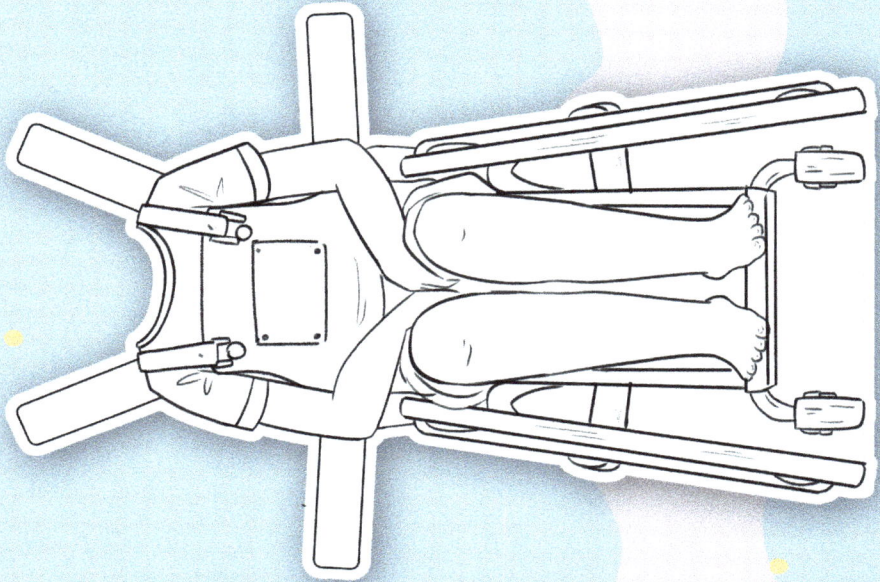

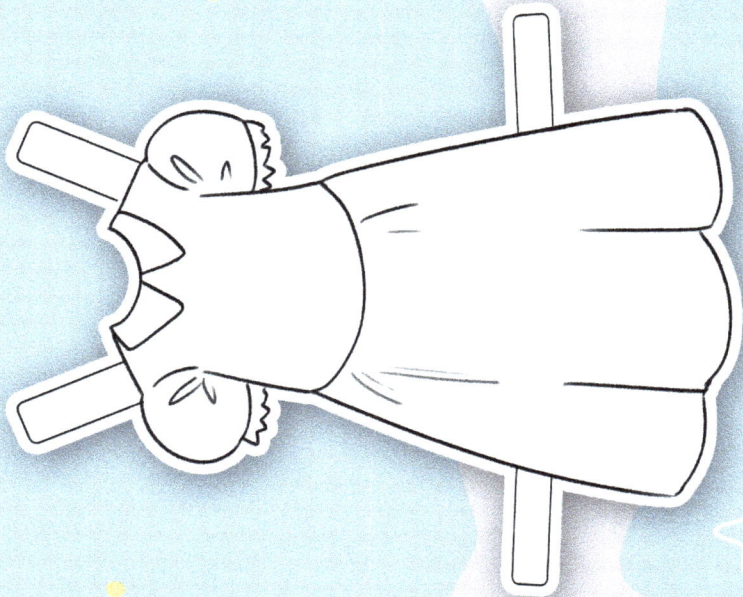

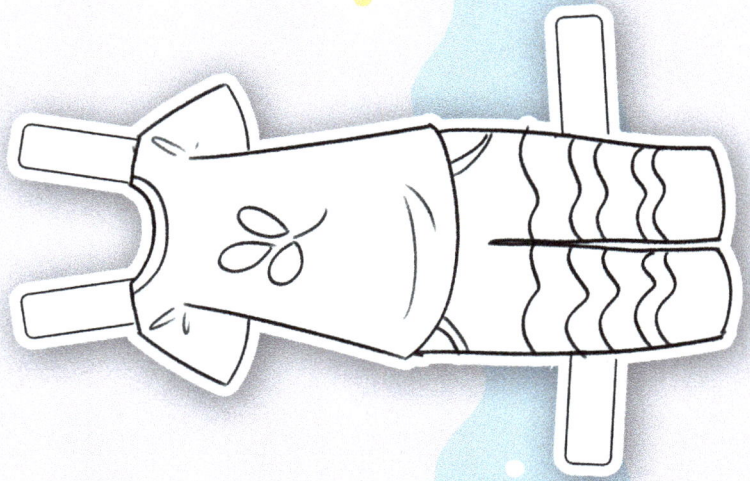

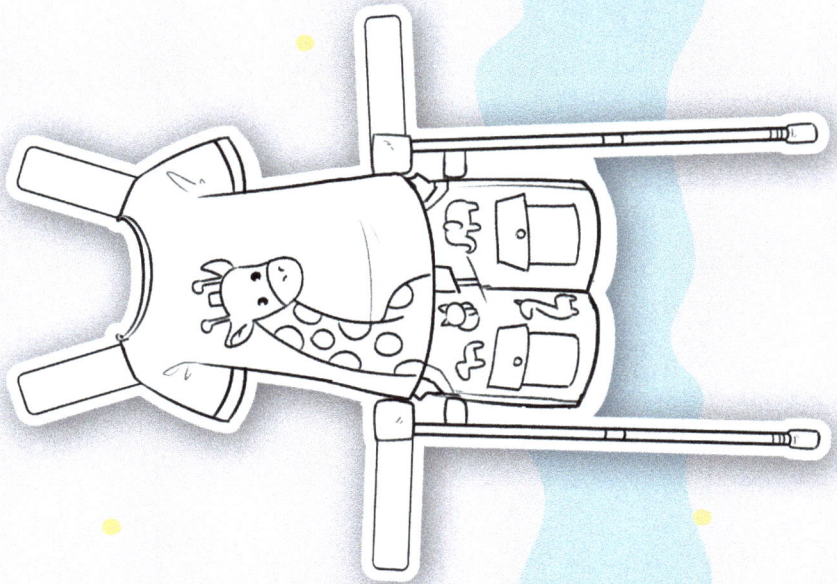

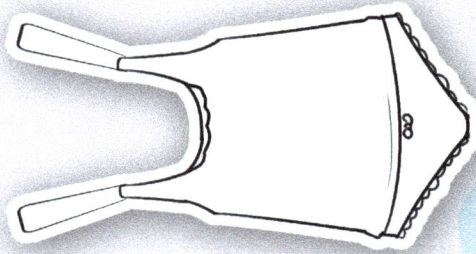

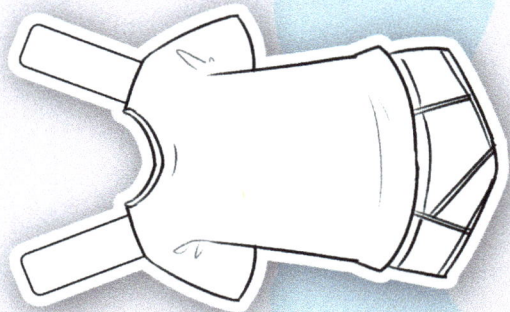

NOTE TO THE READER

These PaperDolls are the perfect resource to facilitate open and honest conversations about bodies and anatomy with your children. Of course, you may still have some reservations and questions regarding these conversations, such as...

Won't talking encourage or increase their curiosity? Kids are naturally curious about bodies and talking to them straight-on helps them to learn about themselves. It satisfies their curiosity, which means they don't need to undertake their own investigations (behind closed doors with another child).

Won't this take away their innocence? Knowing the correct anatomical names for body parts will actually protect your child. It makes them less vulnerable to sexual abuse and gives them the language and ability to clearly communicate when inappropriate touching occurs.

What if they use these words at school, or in a silly way? That's entirely possible! Make sure to let your child know that the names for our genitals are private words and they shouldn't be used in public places, like the park or school. Oh, and in case you were wondering, it's okay to use fun family names for body parts, but it's important that your kids know the correct names too.

I find it too embarrassing. Many parents feel the same. The solution? Start talking when your hands are busy cutting and colouring so you can avoid eye contact with your child. Once you've started, you'll find the conversation gets more relaxed and that subsequent conversations are much easier to start.

I don't know what to say. It's common to feel unsure when starting something new, which is why you'll find ideas for discussions below to help you get started!

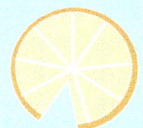

GETTING STARTED

Grab this book, some cardboard (a cereal or biscuit box works), scissors, a glue stick, colouring-in pencils or pens, and tell your child that you have some PaperDolls for them to play with—but first, they'll need to pick which dolls they want to play with! Ask your child to have a look at the PaperDolls and pick two to colour in.

Casually ask your child some questions about the PaperDolls as they colour them; for example, the Doll's name, what they like to do, what colour hair will they have, etc. They may or may not respond.

Use some of the discussion ideas below to start a conversation while your child is colouring, cutting, and playing.

DISCUSSION IDEAS

Here are some ideas for talking to your child. They'll help you work out what your child already knows, how much they've understood, and whether they need more information.

NAMES OF THEIR GENITALS

Grab any naked PaperDoll and, while pointing out the different body parts, ask your child to name them. Tell your child the correct name for the genitals. Male parts are the penis, scrotum, testes or testicles (the squishy bits inside the scrotum), and bottom (or anus). The female parts are the vulva, vagina (inside part), and bottom (or anus).

WHICH BODY PARTS ARE DIFFERENT AND WHY

Grab any male and female PaperDoll and lay them in front of your child. Ask them to point out the body parts that are the same—e.g., the arms, feet, and belly button. Then, ask them to point out the body parts that are different—e.g., the hair and genitals.

Discuss why the genitals are different. Explain that female bodies usually have a vulva and that male bodies usually have a penis and that the parts that are different are what determine a person's biological sex. You could use mums and dads as examples.

Sex (male, female and intersex)

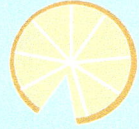

Grab three short-haired PaperDolls: one with a penis, one with a vulva, and one with no genitals. Ask your child if they can point out which parts of the body are different.

It's time to touch upon genitals and sex. Reiterate that the parts that are different are what determine whether you're male, female, or intersex. The male parts are the penis, scrotum and testes (or testicles). The female parts are the vulva, vagina, clitoris, and ovaries. If you're intersex, you don't have solely male or female parts, but have a mix of these parts instead.

Gender (boy, girl, and transgender)

Grab two PaperDolls, one with a penis and one with a vulva.

Pass your child the female PaperDoll and ask them what clothes they should wear. While they are dressing their PaperDoll, dress your male PaperDoll in a dress and explain that your PaperDoll is a girl.

Your child will either accept your statement or disagree. If they disagree and say that your PaperDoll is a boy (not a girl), ask them why they disagree.

If they agree that your PaperDoll is a girl, ask them why they agree. Can someone with a penis be a girl? Or can they only be a boy?

Explain to your child that girls usually have female parts, but not always. Some children with male parts may see themselves as girls, and some children with female parts may see themselves as boys. Remind your child that everyone is different and that's okay.

When a person with male parts sees themselves as a girl, they are a transgender girl, and when a person with female parts sees themselves as a boy, they are a transgender boy.

GENDER STEREOTYPES

Grab two short-haired PaperDolls, one with a penis and one with a vulva. Dress the female PaperDoll in something feminine and the male PaperDoll in something masculine.

Point to a dressed PaperDoll and ask your child whether the PaperDoll is boy or a girl. Once your child answers, ask why they are a boy or girl. How can they tell? By their clothing or hair? By the toys they play with?

Swap the clothing on the PaperDolls and ask whether it's okay for a boy to wear a dress, to like the colour pink, or to play with a PaperDoll. Then ask whether it's okay for a girl to like playing with toy trucks and to wear pants instead of a dress.

Explain to your child that gender (e.g., boy and girl) is about how people expect you to act. So, people may expect a girl to have long hair and a boy to have short hair. We call this a stereotype, because we think we know who that person is by how they look, what they wear, and the toys they play with. Stereotypes are silly and we don't need to follow them. Regardless of what body parts you have, it is okay for you to have long or short hair, to wear what you want, and to play with whichever toys you want.

SAME-SEX RELATIONSHIPS

Grab the wedding clothes and ask your child which PaperDolls could get married. If they select a male and female PaperDoll, ask them if two males (or boys) or two females (or girls) could get married. Listen to their answer, and explain that when they grow up, they may fall in love with someone of the opposite sex, the same sex, or no one at all. Discuss the different values surrounding same-sex relationships within your faith or community.

PRIVATE PARTS

Grab two PaperDolls, one with a penis and one with a vulva. Ask your child to name and point to the private parts of the body. (The private parts of the body are the vulva/vagina, penis, scrotum/testicles, nipples, bottom/anus, and also the mouth. The mouth is included because sexual abuse can involve a child's mouth.)

Explain that the private parts of the body are the parts that are covered by our underwear or swimming clothes, as well as the mouth. These parts of the body are private because they are just for you. This means that no one should touch or look at these parts without your permission. We have these rules to keep kids safe.

Ask your child to dress their PaperDoll so their private parts are covered.

BODY SAFETY

Grab a dressed male and female PaperDoll and tell your child that they are friends. It is a hot day, so they want to play outside with the garden hose. Undress both PaperDolls and explain that, since they don't want to get their clothes wet, you'll have to take their clothes off. One PaperDoll notices that the other PaperDoll has private parts that are different to their own. They ask if they can have a look (or touch them).

Ask your child what the other PaperDoll should do.

Explain to your child that that they are the boss of their body and that no one can touch or look at their private parts without their permission. Tell them that it is not okay for a person to ask to look at or touch their private parts (or for them to look at and touch another person's private parts).

Discuss different scenarios with your child.

What if they say no, and the other PaperDoll doesn't listen? What if they touch the PaperDoll's private parts without asking first? What could the PaperDoll do? Who could they tell? How could they stop them?

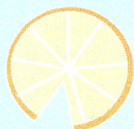

Or, what if the PaperDoll said yes and allowed the other PaperDoll to look at or touch their private parts? Are they breaking your family rules about touching private parts?

Discuss what they could do if someone wanted to touch or look at their private parts. What should they do? Who should they tell? What if the person who asked said it was a secret? Who is allowed to touch someone else's private parts, and in what situations?

NUDITY

Grab a PaperDoll and tell your child that you want to dress your PaperDoll to go shopping. Ask them what clothes they should wear and whether they can go to the shops with no clothes on (naked). When your child says they can't, ask why.

Share your family rules about nudity—i.e., when and where is it acceptable for someone to be naked? Explain that we have rules about our bodies that keep them safe. Discuss different scenarios where nudity might or might not be appropriate. Can they be naked if they are playing in the back yard? What about if they had friends over to play? Or what if there was a stranger in the yard, chopping down a tree? Could they be naked, or would they need to wear clothes?

ABOUT THE AUTHOR

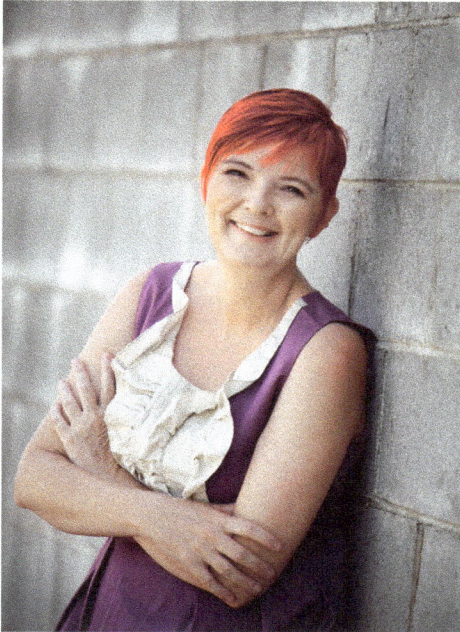

CATH HAKANSON has been talking to clients about sex for the past 25 years as a nurse, midwife, sex therapist, researcher, author and educator. She's spent the past 11 years trying to unravel why parents (herself included) struggle with sex education. Her solution was to create Sex Ed Rescue, an online resource that simplifies sex education and helps parents to empower their children with the right information about sex, so kids can talk to them about anything, no matter what.

Cath has lived all over Australia but currently lives in Perth with her partner, 2 children, and ever-growing menagerie of pets. Despite having an unusual profession, she bakes, sews, and knits for sanity, collects sexual trivia, and tries really hard not to embarrass her children in public. Well, most of the time anyway!

If you'd like to know more, please visit her online home at

SexEdRescue.com

www.ingramcontent.com/pod-product-compliance
Lightning Source LLC
Chambersburg PA
CBHW041101050426
42334CB00063B/3280